20/20 Diet Recipes: Recipes to help you Lose weight Were Other Diets Fail.

by Jessy Smith

Copyright © 2014 by: Jessy Smith

All rights reserved. This book or any portion thereof may not be reproduced or used in any manner whatsoever without the express written permission of the publisher except for the use of brief quotations in a book review.

Disclaimer:
The information provided in this book is designed to provide helpful information on the subjects discussed. The publisher and author are not responsible for any specific health or allergy needs that may require medical supervision and are not liable for any damages or negative consequences from any treatment, action, application or preparation, to any person reading or following the information in this book.

Table of Contents
Introduction -   -   -   -   -   -   -   -   - 5
Phase 1: The 5 Day Boost   -   -   -   -   -   -   - 9
    Ultimate Green Tea
    Apple, Lemon Juice & Cinnamon
    Pistachio nuts, Eggs & Lemon juice
    Almond Crackers
    Baked Walnut-Cinnamon Apples
    Almond Coconut Pancakes
    Almond Macaroons
    Apple wonders
    Apple & Raisin Slaw
    Apple Butter
    DIJON Mustard & CHICKEN Breast
    Garlic-Citrus Grilled Chicken
    Scrambled Hard-boiled eggs with Walnuts
    Raisin Omelet
    Savoring Sautéed Kale
Phase II: The 5 Day Sustain   -   -   -   -   -   - 25
    Delicious Carrot Salad
    Delicious Fruit Crumble
    Fantastic Fruity loops
    Quick Apple Breakfast
    Avocado with Pan Seared Salmon
    Special Apple Oatmeal
    Cayenne Citrus Marinade with Grilled Cod
    Tasty Chicken Marinade
    Blueberry Candies
    Delicious Granola
    Mushrooms with Baked Cod
    Blueberry Walnut Pancakes
    20/20 Carrot Cake
    Apple Allure Smoothie
    Grilled Lemon Chicken
Phase III: The 20 Day Attain -   -   -   -   -   - -- 41
    Brown Apple Treat
    Dijon Steak
    Italian Marinated Chicken
    Vegetables & Baked Salmon
    Shrimp Stuffed Avocados

    Fantastic Fruity Chicken
    Spiced Chicken with Pineapple Sauce
    Almond Asparagus
    Cinnamon Carrots
    Garlic Mushrooms and Chili
    Mushroom Salad
    Watercress and Walnut Salad
    Ultimate Almond Milk
    Pita Bread and Hummus
    Tasty Walnut Cookies

The 20 Key Foods To Eat - - - - - - - 57
Foods & Allergies - - - - - - - - 59
Bonus Recipes - - - - - - - - 60
    Flourless Pie Crust
    Almond Chicken Salad
    Creamy Almond Milk
    Appetizing Coconut Bread
    Chestnut Cake
    Apple Cinnamon Turnover
    Favorite Spinach Fritata
    Broiled Cod with Ginger
    Salmon and Zucchini Fritters
    Lime Shrimp
    Chicken Fast Fingers
    Broccoli with Basil Mushrooms

Enjoy - - - - - - - - - 74
Other Health and Fitness Book - - - - - 75

Introduction

The 20/20 diet is a conservative plan created by Dr. Phil to help change the way we eat in order to give our body the best resources to enable it function properly. It is a guide to using the latest scientific research to plan your own personal strategy for success in losing weight. According to Dr. Phil, diet fail because of "The Seven Ugly Truth" about dieting which he calls blunders. This diets makes you feel hungry, thereby making you crave for more food. Also, this other diets make you feel restricted in what you can eat-causing you to "rebel" against the diet.

Once we understand why diets fail, we can use the latest scientific studies to help create our own meal plan. The 20/20 Plan is a combination of sensible exercise with some very special foods—Dr. Phil calls these the "20/20" foods. The foods in the 20/20 Diet are (naturally) called "20/20 Foods." They are selected because they help to boost your metabolism--that's called the body's "thermogenesis." Also, these foods tends to make you feel full and satisfied when you eat them. Finally, this feeling full effect last a longer time than with other foods.

Dr. Phil believes that being overweight is not because you use food normally--it's because you MISUSE food. He believes that one main reason for the 20/20 diet is to help increase your metabolism. His diet consist of 20 key foods that would help you succeed in your weight loss were other Diet fail. He has written a book that includes the phases of the diet, along with recipes. Below we will review those phases and then include a collection of recipes for each phase to help you succeed in this Diet.

The 20/20 Diet plan Includes three Phases:

PHASE I - THE 5 DAY BOOST: This Phase allow your body to adjust to the new dietary balance. This keeps you on the right track, and is mostly a beginner phase, so you can better understand your body's signals about hunger versus habit.

PHASE II - THE 5 DAY SUSTAIN: This Phase Builds on the success of the first phase by adding some more 20/20 foods to the mix, which offers more nutritional benefits, and give you the range of vitamins and minerals your body needs.

PHASE III - THE 20 DAY ATTAIN: In this phase your goal is to maintain the steady weight loss, and even add some dining out occasions. There are more foods to choose from.

The 20/20 Diet is designed to Jump-start your weight loss and help you succeed were other diet fail.

When to Eat

You eat every four hours spaced according to the time you wake up, which results in about four meals a day.

Breakfast at 6:00am

Snack at 10:00am

Lunch at 2:00pm

Dinner at 6:00pm

OR

Breakfast at 8:00am

Lunch at 12:00pm

Snack at 4:00pm

Dinner at 8:00pm

OR

Breakfast at 9:00am

Lunch at 1:00pm

Snack at 5:00pm

Dinner at 9:00pm

Side Note:

The purpose of this recipe book is to help as many people as possible stick to their diets and reach their health goals. That's why we have worked so hard to prepare this 20/20 diet recipes. The Only thing we ask for is that you recommend and give us honest review on amazon. If you think the recipes are good, then let everyone know about it. We Appreciate You.

Now On to the Recipes:

Phase 1: The 5 Day Boost

In the 5 Day Boost Phase, you will find meals and Snacks and green tea. This phase consist of the 20 key foods that would jump start your weight loss. By following this Plan the person get fuller and never craves for more food. Also, In this Phase you are advised to drink a lot of water, because often times we confuse being thirsty with being hunger. Studies shows that water actually increases metabolism.

Ultimate Green Tea

Green tea is a great alternative for people who are on weight loss programs because it can help them lead a healthier lifestyle. For instance, instead of drinking coffee and cream which are high in calories, green tea can not only save you from taking in too much calories but also let you take in several healthful substances like polyphenols and flavonoids. Green tea also contains a small amount of caffeine, a key substance used in weight loss because of its appetite-suppressant properties.

Ingredients:

1 Anjou pear, chopped
1/4 cup white raisins (or dried mulberries)
1 teaspoon freshly minced gingerroot
1 large handful chopped romaine lettuce
1 tablespoon hemp seeds
1 cup unsweetened brewed green tea, cooled
7 to 9 ice cubes

How you make it:

1. Place all the ingredients except the ice in a Blender, and process until smooth and creamy.
2. Add ice if desired and process again.
3. Serve and Drink chilled.

Apple, Lemon Juice & Cinnamon

Ingredients:

6 apples
Greek yogurt (made with real sugar, not artificial sweetener)
2-3 Tbsp. lemon juice
Cinnamon

How you make it:

1. Mix Greek Yogurt and lemon juice. Core and slice apples.
2. Mix with honey and blend all until smooth. Sprinkle with cinnamon and serve.

Pistachio nuts, Eggs & Lemon juice

Ingredients:

3 hard-boiled egg yolks
1 cup olive oil
Sea salt and pepper
1/2 of lemon juice
1 ½ Tbsp. basil, finely chopped
3 Tbsp. parsley, finely chopped
3 Tbsp. ground pistachio nuts

How you make it:

1. Whisk hard-boiled egg yolks in a bowl. Continue to whisk and pour in oil in a very slow trickle, until it has all been absorbed. Still whisking, add sea salt, pepper and lemon juice to taste.
2. Stir through basil, parsley and nuts to give a smooth very thick sauce.
3. If the mayonnaise curdles, continue its preparation to the finish.
4. Beat another hard-boiled egg yolk in a clean bowl and gradually whisk in the curdled sauce. The mayonnaise keeps, covered and chilled, for up to 24 hours.
5. It is less successful if made with a food processor or blender. Yield: about 1 cup.

Almond Crackers

Ingredients:

Unsalted almonds, ground into a flour
1 Tbsp. olive oil or coconut oil
Sea salt
Water

How you make it:

1. Combine almond flour, sea salt, oil and enough water to bind it together.
2. Pat out on a cookie sheet lined with parchment paper. Bake at 300-350 F until crispy.

Baked Walnut-Cinnamon Apples

Ingredients:

4 small apples
1 cup raisins
1/4 tsp. cinnamon
1/2 tsp. vanilla
1/2 cup water
1/4 cup walnuts

How you make it:

1. Heat oven to 375 F. Core and piece apples with a fork in several places around the center, to prevent them from bursting.
2. Mix raisins, nuts, cinnamon, and vanilla in a small bowl.
3. Fill center of each apple with this mixture. Place in a glass-baking dish and pour water into pan.
4. Cover with foil and bake about 30 minutes or until tender.

Almond Coconut Pancakes

Ingredients:

1 hard-boiled egg
1/4 cup of ground almonds
1/4 cup of coconut milk
Cook as regular pancakes in coconut or olive oil.

How you make it:

1. To cook an oven pancake: Preheat oven.
2. Heat the pan (a cast iron frying pan works the best) in a 425 F oven until hot, add some olive oil or coconut oil to the pan (1 Tbsp.) and then add the hard-boiled egg mixture. Cook for 10 minutes. No turning.
3. It will not puff up like the ones made with rice flour instead of almonds.

Almond Macaroons

Ingredients:

1-1/4 cup almonds (Unsalted, Dry Roasted)
1/8 tsp. cinnamon
2 Tbsp. grated lemon peel
2 hard-boiled egg whites, beaten
1/4 cup raw honey
2 Tbsp. lemon juice

How you make it:

1. Grind almonds coarsely. Combine cinnamon and lemon and add.
2. Beat hard-boiled egg whites very stiff, fold in honey and continue beating.
3. Fold in lemon juice with almond mixture and blend.
4. Drop from a tsp. onto ungreased parchment paper.
5. Bake 30 minutes at 250 F. Remove from paper while still slightly warm. Makes 30 macaroons.

Apple wonders

Apple is a great fruit that taste really well when used in making smoothie. It has wonderful flavors, which makes drinking green smoothies an ultimate delight.

Ingredients:

4 cups of kale
4 small apples
½ lemon juice
1 cup ice

How you make it:

1. First, Place the kale and water into blender and blend until mixture is a green juice-like consistency.
2. Stop blender and add the other remaining ingredients and blend.
3. Add ice if desired and blend again until creamy.

Apple & Raisin Slaw

Ingredients:

1 large tart green apple (such as Granny Smith), cored, coarsely chopped
5 cups coarsely chopped green cabbage (about 1/2 medium head)
1 cup coarsely grated carrots (about 2 medium)
1/2 cup raisins
5 cups coarsely chopped red cabbage (about 1/2 medium head)
1/2 cup raw unsalted sunflower seeds, toasted
1/2 cup chopped fresh dill or 3 tablespoons dried dill weed
2 tablespoons Olive oil
2 tablespoons apple cider vinegar
1 1/2 cups plain nonfat Greek yogurt

How you make it:

1. Combine cabbages, carrots, apple, raisins and sunflower seeds in very large bowl.
2. Whisk yogurt, dill, Olive oil and vinegar in medium bowl to blend.
3. Add dressing to cabbage mixture and toss to coat.
4. Season to taste with salt and pepper. (Can be prepared 3 hours ahead. Cover and refrigerate.)

Apple Butter

Ingredients:

- 6 pounds cooking apples
- 6 cups apple juice
- 3 cups sugar
- ½ teaspoon ground cloves
- 2 teaspoons cinnamon
- 1 teaspoon fresh lemon juice

How you make it:

1. Core and thinly slice apples into a large heavy saucepan.
2. Add apple juice and cook until soft, about 30 minutes.
3. Pour apples into a large sieve and press until all fruit passes through and leaves skin.
4. Discard skin. Repeat process until all apples are sieved.
5. Return pulp to the heavy saucepan and boil gently, stirring frequently, until thick.
6. Stir in sugar, spices, and lemon juice. Cook, stirring over low heat about 1 hour.
7. Pour into sterilized 1/2 pint jars leaving 1/4 inch headspace; adjust lids and process in a boiling water bath for 10 minutes after water comes to a boil. You can successfully make half this recipe if desired. Make 8 - 1/2 pints.

DIJON Mustard & CHICKEN Breast

Ingredients:

1 lb. chicken breast
Marinade for several hours in:
5 tbs. Dijon Mustard (grainy)
1/4 cup Fat Free Italian Dressing

How you make it:

1. Let your chicken breast sit for several hours in mixture.
2. Preheat GFG and wipe with Olive Oil.
3. Cook chicken on hot grill until juices run clear --- turn once while cooking.

Garlic-Citrus Grilled Chicken

Ingredients:

4 lb. Boneless skinless Chicken Breasts
2 tsp. Lime Zest
3/4 cup fresh Lemon Juice
3/4 cup fresh Lime Juice
1 1/2 Tbs. Granulated Sugar
2 tsp. Lemon Zest
2 tsp. Garlic, minced
1/4 tsp. Cayenne Pepper
1/4 cup Olive Oil

How you make it:

1. In a small saucepan, whisk the lemon and lime zests and juices with the sugar, minced garlic, and cayenne pepper.
2. Warm for about 5 minutes, until the sugar is dissolved. Whisk in the oil.
3. Remove from the stove and let the marinade cool.
4. Arrange the chicken breasts in a large dish.
5. Try to set it up so the chicken is in a single layer. Prick the meat in several places with a fork, and pour the marinade over the top.
6. Let the chicken marinate, covered and chilled, for at least 3 hours, turning once. (You may opt to marinate the chicken overnight, if you prefer.)
7. Using tongs, transfer the chicken to an oiled preheated grill.
8. Baste the chicken with the marinade and turn the meat at least 3 times while cooking, basting each time you turn.
9. Grill until chicken is cooked through.

Scrambled Hard-boiled eggs with Walnuts

Ingredients:

3 hard-boiled eggs
1/2 cup chopped basil
1/3 cup chopped walnuts
Pepper

How you make it:

1. Whisk hard-boiled eggs in a bowl then place in a frying pan on medium heat, stirring continuously.
2. When hard-boiled eggs have almost cooked through, add the basil and continue cooking for another minute, or until hard-boiled eggs are cooked through.
3. Pepper to taste. Remove from heat and stir in walnuts before serving.

Raisin Omelet

Ingredients:

2 Tbsp. raisins
3 hard-boiled eggs
Dash ground cinnamon
Dash ground allspice
Dash nutmeg

How you make it:

2. Boil raisins in water for 1 minute. Drain well. In a bowl, beat together hard-boiled eggs, cinnamon, all spice and nutmeg.
3. Stir in raisins. Heat a frying pan lined with baking paper. Pour the beaten hard-boiled eggs onto the baking paper.
4. When the bottom of the hard-boiled eggs have cooked, turn the mixture over by placing another sheet of baking paper to the side and flipping and hard-boiled eggs onto it, then transfer it onto the heated frying pan and cook for another 2-3 minutes, or until browned on the bottom.

Savoring Sautéed Kale

Ingredients:

1 lb. kale trimmed and chopped
1 Tbsp. olive oil
2 Tbsp. walnuts, lightly toasted
1 large garlic clove, crushed
2 Tbsp. lemon juice

How you make it:

2. Cook the kale in a large pot of boiling water until tender (about 10 minutes); drain well.
3. Coat a large skillet with oil. Sauté garlic over medium heat until just golden (about 3 minutes).
4. Add kale to skillet. Stir in the olive oil, sauté until heated through (about 5 minutes).
5. Stir in pine nuts, remove skillet from heat. Sprinkle kale mixture with lemon juice.
6. Transfer to a shallow serving dish and serve immediately.

Phase II: The 5 Day Sustain

In this 5 Days Sustain Plan, you would find Meals, snacks and Smoothies, which offers more nutritional benefits, and would give you the range of vitamins and minerals your body needs. You would find out that each meals includes two of the 20/20 Foods as well as some protein source. The four Hours Spacing Per Meals still applies here.

Delicious Carrot Salad

Ingredients:

1 lb. shredded carrots
20 oz. pineapple
8 oz. coconut milk
¾ cup flaked coconut
¾ cup raisins
2 Tbsp. raw honey

How you make it:

Combine all ingredients, tossing well. Cover and chill.

Delicious Fruit Crumble

Ingredients:

1/2 cup frozen blueberries
1/4 cup prunes or dates
1/2 cup almond flour
1 cup walnuts or pecans
1/2 tsp. cinnamon
Real Sugar (Not artificial sweetener)

How you make it:

2. Preheat the oven to 350 F. Place your fruit of choice in an oven safe dish of the appropriate size. Puree the prunes or date in a food processor along with the almond flour.
3. Add the whole nuts and cinnamon and pulse briefly to combine. Taste and adjust sweetness with sugar.
4. The mixture should hold together when you squeeze it, but be crumbly if you rub it between your fingers. If it is too dry add, a little splash of juice; if it is too wet, add some more nuts.
5. Press the nut mixture down firmly over the fruit. Place in the oven and bake for 30 minutes.
6. Let cool for 15 minutes before eating. Then refrigerates well for at least one day and reheated for breakfast. Serves 3-4.

Fantastic Fruity loops

Ingredients:

2 ¾ Small apples
2 cup strawberries
1 tsp. cinnamon
1/4 cup purified water.

How you make it:

1. Clean, core and chop apples. Add chopped apples and strawberries in a blender and add a 1/4 cup of purified water and cinnamon and process about 30 seconds or until smooth.
2. Pour mixture on a Teflex sheet (a Teflon-coated sheet commonly used to dehydrate delicate foods) and place in a plastic dehydrator.
3. Dehydrate for 6-8 hours, remove sheet and flip fruit. Continue drying another 4-6 hours or until desired consistency is achieved.
4. Use a pizza cutter to slice into snack-size pieces. This recipe may also be done in an oven. A good rule of thumb when using an oven to dehydrate is to set the temperature between 100 and 150 F and keep the oven slightly cracked for the duration of the dehydration.

Quick Apple Breakfast

Ingredients:

1 large apple, chopped into bite sized pieces
1 medium carrot, grated
Cinnamon to taste
Handful of raisins

How you make it:

Mix the apple, carrot, and raisins in a bowl, sprinkle cinnamon over the top.

Avocado with Pan Seared Salmon

Ingredients:

2 large avocados, cut and peeled
3 Tbsp. freshly squeezed lime juice (can substitute lemon)
3-4 Tbsp. olive oil
1 Tbsp. minced shallots or green onion
1 Tbsp. minced parsley
Sea salt and pepper to taste
1 ½ lbs. of salmon fillets

How you make it:

1. Put avocado pieces and lime juice into a food processor or blender and pulse until blended.
2. Slowly add olive oil, pulsing, until you reach desired consistency of sauce.
3. Add minced shallots (or green onions) and parsley, pulse just until combined.
4. Remove to a bowl, salt and pepper to taste.
5. Coat the bottom of a sauté pan with oil, heat on medium high until almost smoking. Season both sides of the salmon fillets with salt and pepper.
6. Place the salmon into the pan, skin side down. Cook the salmon until about medium doneness, about 3-4 minutes per side. Serve salmon with avocado sauce. Serves 4.

Special Apple Oatmeal

A delicious and warming breakfast treat

Ingredients:

1/2 cup chopped apple
3 cups apple juice
1/2 tsp ground cinnamon
1/4 cup maple syrup
1/4 cup raisins
1 1/2 cups quick oats
1/4 cup chopped walnuts

How you make it:

1. Combine apple juice and cinnamon in a medium saucepan.
2. Bring to a boil.
3. Stir in oats, chopped apple, maple syrup and raisins.
4. Reduce heat and cook until most of juice is absorbed, stirring occasionally.
5. Fold in walnuts. Serve.

Cayenne Citrus Marinade with Grilled Cod

Ingredients:

1/4 cup orange juice
1 1/2 Tbsp. lemon juice
3 Tbsp. lime juice
1/8 tsp. cayenne pepper
2 Tbsp. olive oil
1 lb. cod fillets
2 Tbsp. finely chopped chives
1 Tbsp. finely chopped thyme
2 minced garlic cloves

How you make it:

2. Combine orange, lemon and lime juices in a bowl with cayenne pepper, garlic, olive oil, and 1/3 cup of water to make the marinade.
3. Place fish in a flat dish, pour in the marinade, and marinate the fish 15 minutes.
4. Light grill and add the fish. Grill fish 3-4 minutes per side, basting often with the marinade.
5. Serve the fish with a spoonful of marinade and sprinkle with chives and thyme.

Tasty Chicken Marinade

Ingredients:

1/2 cup lime juice
1/4 cup olive oil
3 garlic cloves, minced
1 jalapeno pepper, cut in 1/8 inch slices (do not remove seeds)
1/4 cup chopped cilantro
Dash pepper

How you make it:

1. Combine all ingredients. Pour over one lb. skinless/boneless chicken breast halves.
2. Marinate at least 2 hours. Remove chicken from marinade and either grill or broil.
3. Brush with remaining marinade during cooking.

Blueberry Candies

Ingredients:

5 cup blueberries
4 tsp. cinnamon
1 tsp. vanilla extract
1 1/2 tsp. ginger
2 hard-boiled egg whites
1/4 cup raw honey

How you make it:

1. In a large bowl, whisk hard-boiled egg whites until frothy. Add in honey and vanilla and stir until combined. With a slotted spoon, add blueberries to the hard-boiled egg mixture.
2. Remove and roll in a small bowl filled with a mixture of cinnamon and ginger.
3. Repeat until all blueberries are covered. Using the same slotted spoon, transfer the coated blueberries onto a plastic dehydrator tray.
4. Dehydrate for 24 hours or until dry. After 8-12 hours, or when one side is dry enough, turn them over to dry other side.
5. Serve or store in an airtight container.

Delicious Granola

Ingredients:

1 cup sunflower seeds
6 cups whole wheat or whole grain cereal
2 cup raisins
10 Ziploc bags
1 cup coconut

How you make it:

1. Mix all the ingredients in a bowl and serve 1 cup per day in a Ziploc bag.
2. Be creative for other things to add. Try dried fruit, nuts, etc.

Mushrooms with Baked Cod

Ingredients:

1 pound sliced mushrooms
3 pounds cod fillets
1/2 cup heavy cream
1/2 teaspoon salt
1/4 teaspoon ground black pepper
6 scallions, chopped
1/2 teaspoon Paprika

How You Make It:

1. Arrange fish fillets in single layer in greased 9 by 13 inch pan.
2. Sprinkle with pepper and salt.
3. Stir mushrooms, green onions and cream together in bowl.
4. Spoon over fillets.
5. Bake uncovered in 350 for about 20 minutes, until fish flakes when tested with a fork.
6. Sprinkle with paprika.

Blueberry Walnut Pancakes

Ingredients:

1/2 cup finely ground walnuts (should look like a coarse flour)
Dash of sea salt
1/2 tsp. baking powder (no aluminum)
1 whole organic hard-boiled egg
1/2 cup pure water
1 ½ tsp. olive oil
Chopped walnuts
Blueberries

How you make it:

1. You can vary the ingredients, but make sure the batter is thick enough to support the blueberries and chopped walnuts.
2. Cook each pancake in a little oil, flip once and serve. Can add a small amount of warm, raw honey.

20/20 Carrot Cake

Ingredients:

6 hard-boiled eggs, separated
1/2 cup honey (or less)
1 1/2 cup carrots, cooked and pureed
1 Tbsp. grated orange rind
1 Tbsp. frozen orange juice
3 cup almond flour

How you make it:

1. Preheat oven to 325 F. Beat the hard-boiled egg yolks and honey together. Mix in carrot puree, orange rind, orange juice, and almond flour.
2. Beat the hard-boiled egg whites until stiff and fold in.
3. Spoon into a greased loose-bottomed 9-inch spring form pan.
4. Bake for about 50 minutes or until a skewer inserted into the center of the cake comes out clean.
5. Cool in the pan for 15 minutes, then turn out onto a wire rack to cool completely.
6. Anything could be put in place of the carrots (pumpkin, zucchini, etc.) since the vegetable is pureed first.

Apple Allure Smoothie

This smoothie is simply smooth and classic. You know what they say; "An apple a day keeps the doctor away!" You'll have no problem meeting your daily apple quote with this delicious apple smoothie.

Ingredients:

1 frozen banana, cut into bite-sized pieces
1 organic Granny Smith apple, cored and chopped
(Keep the skin on)
1 tablespoon fresh lemon juice
1 large handful baby spinach
1 cup cold water
2 to 3 pitted dates
1/2 teaspoon cinnamon
1/8 teaspoon nutmeg
4 to 5 ice cubes

How you make it:

2. Place all the ingredients except the ice in a blender, and blend until smooth and creamy.
3. Add the ice and process again. Drink chilled.

Grilled Lemon Chicken

Ingredients:

1/2 tsp. grated lemon peel
1 tbs. olive oil
2 cloves garlic -- crushed (2 to 3)
1 tsp. dried oregano
4 boneless, skinless chicken breast halves (pounded to about 1/2 inch thick)
2 tbs. lemon juice

How you make it:

1. Combine all marinade ingredients. Add chicken breast halves to the marinade.
2. Marinate in the refrigerator for at least 2 hours.
3. Grill until done approximately 8-10 minutes. Make sure the grill is at its hottest while cooking the chicken breasts.

Phase III: The 20 Day Attain

In This Diet Plan you would be adding more healthy foods to your diet. Your aim is to maintain the weight loss. Now you should be seeing New Changes in the way you look. The Meals below would help you maintain the weight loss and keep the fat off while boosting your Metabolism.

Brown Apple Treat

Ingredients:

1/4 teaspoon Dijon Mustard
3 pounds cooking apples
10 slices of bread, cubed (about 4-cups)
1/8 teaspoon sea salt
1/2 cup butter or margarine, melted
3/4 cup brown sugar
1/2 teaspoon cinnamon

How you make it:

1. Wash, peel and core the apples, cut into eighths; place in bottom on crock.
2. In a small bowl combine bread cubes, mustard, salt, sugar, cinnamon, butter; toss together.
3. Place on top of apples. Cover. Cook on low setting 2 to 4 hours.

Dijon Steak

Ingredients:

4 cloves garlic, minced
1 tsp. olive oil
1 tsp. dried basil
2 Tbsp. Dijon mustard
1 tsp. dried thyme
4 rib eye steaks, cut 1 inch thick

How you make it:

1. Sauté garlic and half the oil 2 minutes in a saucepan over high heat.
2. Stir in next 3 ingredients and salt and pepper to taste.
3. Spread mixture over both sides of steaks.
4. Preheat grill machine. Brush remaining oil over both grilling surfaces.
5. Arrange steaks on hot grill, in batches if necessary.

Close cover and cook about 5 minutes, or until meat is cooked thoroughly

Italian Marinated Chicken

Ingredients:

1 can (14 1/2 ounce) Seasoned Chicken Broth with Italian Herbs
6 boneless chicken breast halves

How you make it:

1. Pour broth into shallow non-metallic dish. Add chicken and turn to coat.
2. Cover and refrigerate 30 minutes.
3. Remove chicken from broth. Grill on preheated GFG for 6 to 8 minutes.

Vegetables & Baked Salmon

Ingredients:

1 pound whole mushrooms
1 head cauliflower
2 cloves garlic, grated
2 green peppers
2 teaspoons olive oil
1 red pepper
1/2 teaspoon salt
1 teaspoon crushed dried rosemary leaves
1/4 teaspoon ground black pepper
2 pound salmon fillets
1 tablespoon white vinegar.

How You Make It:

1. Separate the cauliflower into florets. Steam for a minute.
2. Drain thoroughly.
3. Seed peppers, cut into one-inch squares.
4. Clean mushrooms; trim ends.
5. In a large baking dish, combine peppers, mushrooms, cauliflower, rosemary and garlic.
6. Toss with olive oil. Bake at 400° for 15-20 minutes, until vegetables are crisp-tender.
7. Cut salmon into one-inch chunks.
8. Add to vegetable mixture. Return to oven and bake an additional 10-12 minutes, until fish flakes easily with fork.
9. Sprinkle fish mixture with vinegar, salt, and pepper. Toss lightly.

Shrimp Stuffed Avocados

Ingredients:

3 medium size avocados
2 Tbsp. lemon juice
1 1/2 lb. small or medium sized shrimp, cooked, shelled, deveined and chilled

How you make it:

Cut avocados in half; remove seed and skin. Stuff with shrimp. Add lemon juice.

Fantastic Fruity Chicken

Ingredients:

6 Tbsp. olive oil
1 medium onion, chopped
1 garlic clove, minced
2 medium apples, cored and chopped
1/4 cup raisins
1/4 cup finely chopped celery
1/4 cup chopped walnuts
1 hard-boiled egg, beaten
8 large chicken thighs
1 tsp dried tarragon

How you make it:

1. In a medium size frying pan, heat 2 Tbsp. oil. Add onion, celery and garlic.
2. Sauté about 3 minutes, until onion and celery are tender.
3. Remove from heat and add apple, raisins, walnuts, and hard-boiled eggs. Mix well.
4. Preheat oven to 350 F. Prepare chicken thighs by pulling the skin away from the meat without removing it.
5. Stuff apple mixture between the skin and meat. Arrange chicken pieces in a foil-lined 13x9x2 baking dish.
6. In a small bowl, combine the remaining 4 Tbsp. olive oil with tarragon. Brush over chicken thighs.
7. Bake, uncovered, basting every 15 minutes, for 1 hour, until chicken is tender.

Spiced Chicken with Pineapple Sauce

Ingredients:

1 3-lb. chicken, cut up
1 8-oz. can crushed pineapple
1 cup orange juice
1/2 cup raisins
1/2 cup sliced almonds
1/4 tsp. cinnamon
1/4 tsp. ground cloves
Pepper
1 lb. of sliced pureed peaches, fresh, or frozen

How you make it:

1. In a large fry pan, combine chicken, pineapple orange juice, raisins, almonds, cinnamon, and cloves.
2. Simmer, partly covered, for 45 minutes, turning chicken occasionally.
3. Add peach puree to pan and stir until well blended.
4. Simmer uncovered 15 minutes longer, until chicken is tender and sauce is slightly thickened.
5. Season with pepper to taste.

Almond Asparagus

Ingredients:

2 lbs. asparagus
2 Tbsp. olive oil
3/4 cup slivered almonds, toasted
1/4 tsp pepper
1 Tbsp. lemon juice

How you make it:

1. Snap off tough ends of asparagus. Cook asparagus in boiling water to cover 3 minutes or until crisp-tender; drain.
2. Plunge asparagus into ice water to stop the cooking process; drain.
3. Add oil to a large skillet over medium heat; add asparagus and sauté 3-5 minutes.
4. Toss asparagus with lemon juice and remaining ingredients.

Cinnamon Carrots

Ingredient:

6 med carrots, thinly sliced
6 T orange juice
1 1/2 tsp olive oil
3/4 tsp ground cinnamon
1 tsp freshly ground black pepper

How you make it:

1. Place the carrots and orange juice in a medium saucepan.
2. Cover and cook over medium-low heat for 6 minutes or until the carrots are tender-crisp.
3. Add the oil, cinnamon, and pepper. Cook for 1 minute, stirring to coat. Serves 4.

Garlic Mushrooms and Chili

Ingredients:

1 cup button mushrooms
3 garlic cloves, chopped
2 Tbsp. olive oil
1/2 tsp ground paprika

How you make it:

1. Place garlic, paprika and oil in a mixing bowl and combine well.
2. Add mushrooms and coat well in olive oil mixture.
3. Place mushrooms in a frying pan, or on a grill on medium-high heat.
4. Cook for 5-8 minutes, or until mushrooms have browned slightly and have started to shrivel.

Mushroom Salad

Ingredients:

2 Tbsp. lemon juice
1 1/2 Tbsp. olive oil
1 lb. mushrooms, thinly sliced
1 minced garlic clove
2 Tbsp. minced parsley
1 tsp chopped oregano
1/4 tsp pepper

How you make it:

1. Combine everything but mushrooms in a medium bowl, beat with a fork to blend.
2. Then add the mushrooms, toss to coat with dressing and serve immediately.

Watercress and Walnut Salad

Ingredients:

1/4 cup olive oil
1 lb. watercress, finely chopped
1/2 cup cooked and finely diced chicken pieces
1/4 cup walnuts, finely chopped
1 large garlic clove
1/4 cup hazelnuts, finely chopped
1/2 tsp. pepper

How you make it:

2. In a heavy 12-inch skillet, heat the olive oil.
3. Cut the garlic in half lengthwise and add it to the oil. Cook for two minutes, stirring constantly.
4. Remove the garlic and discard. Add all the nuts and cook for 5-6 minutes or until they are browned.
5. Add the chicken and pepper. Cook 2-3 minutes.
6. Dry watercress before adding it to the oil.
7. Working fast, toss the watercress into the mixture in the pan, making sure it is well coated and barely heated through. If left too long it loses some of its crispness. Serve immediately.

Ultimate Almond Milk

Ingredients:

1 cup of almonds (unsalted raw or dry-roasted)
4 cup of water
Banana, prunes, or other dried fruit (optional)

How you make it:

1. To activate almonds, soak overnight and then pour off water. The next day, dip the almonds in boiling water, remove from water and peel away skins.
2. Place in a blender with roughly 4 cups of water (less will make the "milk" thicker) and blend until smooth.
3. To sweeten the milk, add half of a banana or a handful of prunes or other dried fruit.

Pita Bread and Hummus

Ingredients:

2 cloves garlic, crushed
1-16 oz. can of chickpeas
3-5 tbsp. Lemon juice (depending on taste)
5 pita bread cut in quarters
1 1/2 tbsp. Tahini
1/2 tsp sea salt
1/4 cup liquid from can of chickpeas
2 tbsp. Olive oil

How You Prepare It:

1. Drain chickpeas and set aside liquid from can.
2. In blender or food processor, combine tahini, lemon juice, garlic and salt.
3. Add one-quarter cup of liquid from chickpeas.
4. Blend until thoroughly mixed and smooth, for 3-5 minutes on low.
5. Place in serving bowl, and create a shallow well in the center of the hummus.
6. Add a small amount (1-2 tbsp.) of olive oil in the well.
7. Serve immediately with fresh, warm or toasted pita bread.

Tasty Walnut Cookies

Ingredients:

2 cup walnuts
1/8 cup raw honey (more or less to taste)
1 Tbsp. cinnamon
2 hard-boiled egg whites, whisked till frothy

How you make it:

1. Grind nuts and cinnamon in blender or food processor.
2. Stir in honey. Combine with hard-boiled egg whites.
3. Drop by tsp on oiled cookie sheet. Bake at 350 F for 15 minutes.
4. Cookies will be soft; do not over bake. Makes 15 cookies. This works well for a pie crust too.

The 20 Key Foods To Eat

Below are the list of the 20 key Foods to Eat in the 5 Day Boost Phase:

Coconut Oil
Green Tea
Mustard (Yellow or Dijon)
Olive Oil
Walnut
Almonds
Apples
Chickpeas
Dried Plums (pumes)
Green (Any Kind of Leafy Green)
Lentils
Peanut butter (natural)
Pistachios (Roasted, Unsalted in the shell)
Raisin
Yogurt (non-Fat)
Eggs
Cod
Rye
Tofu
Whey protein.

Phase Two Foods

Tuna
Chicken Breast
Black bean
Carrot
Tomatoes
Mushroom
Blueberries
Grapes
Oats
Brown rice
Corn
Avocado
Sunflower Seeds
Cashew
Orange

Foods & Allergies

Some of the listed foods are associated with some allergies, intolerance & Sensitivity. So you are free to substitute them with the following related food. This is to help you succeed with this Diet. Also Note that before trying any new food, you should get approval from your doctor before proceeding.

Below are some of The Food and their Substitute:

Food	Substitute
Peanut Butter	Almonds, hazelnut, Sunflower Seeds, pumpkin butters
Walnut	Pumpkin Seeds
Rye Bread	Whole grain bread
Greek Yogurt	Rice milk, Almond Yogurt
Whey Protein	Brown Rice, Hemp Seed, Pea Protein
Eggs	Tofu or Mashed Chickpeas
Fish	Chicken Breast or other lean protein Sources
Tofu	Eggs or Lean protein Chicken breast or chickpeas

Bonus Recipes

Here, In This Bonus Recipes, we have included lots of healthy and delicious recipes, So you can have Variety of recipes to choose from that are in line with the 20/20 Diet plan and would help you live a healthy lifestyle.

Flourless Pie Crust

Ingredients:

1 1/4 cup almond meal
2/3 cup coconut oil
1/4 tsp. sea salt
5 Tbsp. icy water

How you make it:

1. Combine almond flour and sea salt in a mixing bowl, stir in coconut oil and mix until mixture resembles coarse crumbs.
2. Mix in water, 1 Tbsp. at a time, until dough is formed. Refrigerate until ready to use.
3. When ready, roll out and place in a pie dish. Fill your favorite fruit (Apples, blueberries) and bake at 450 F for 15 minutes or until crust turns a rich golden brown.

Almond Chicken Salad

Ingredients:

4 cups cubed cooked chicken
1 cup chopped celery
1 1/2 cups seedless green grapes
3/4 cup sliced green onion
3 free-range hard-boiled eggs, chopped
1/2 cup almond butter
1/2 tsp. pepper
1/4 cup sour cream
1 Tbsp. prepared mustard
1 tsp. Sea salt
1/4 tsp. onion pepper
1/4 tsp. celery salt
1/8 tsp. dry mustard
1/8 tsp. paprika
1 kiwifruit, peeled and sliced (optional)
1/2 cup slivered almonds, toasted

How you prepare it:

1. Combine grapes, celery, onions, chicken, and hard-boiled eggs, in large bowl.

2. Combine the other nine ingredients, in another bowl; stir until smooth.

3. Pour over chicken mixture and toss gently.

4. Stir in almonds and serve immediately, or refrigerate and add almonds right before serving.

5. Garnish with kiwifruit if desired.

Creamy Almond Milk

Ingredients:

1 cup of almonds (unsalted raw or dry-roasted)
4 cup of water
Banana, prunes, or other dried fruit (optional)

How you make it:

4. To activate almonds, soak overnight and then pour off water. The next day, dip the almonds in boiling water, remove from water and peel away skins.
5. Place in a blender with roughly 4 cups of water (less will make the "milk" thicker) and blend until smooth.
6. To sweeten the milk, add half of a banana or a handful of prunes or other dried fruit.

Appetizing Coconut Bread

Ingredients:

2 hard-boiled eggs
1/3 cup olive oil
1/2 cup honey
1 cup coconut milk
1 tsp. 100% vanilla essence
1 cup almond meal
1/2 cup coconut flour
1 tsp. baking powder (or separate 2 hard-boiled eggs and beat the hard-boiled egg whites until stiff peaks form, then fold into the coconut mixture to help in aerating the bread)
1/4 c desiccated coconut

How you make it:

1. Preheat oven to 350 F. Cream hard-boiled eggs, oil, and honey in a large bowl until light and fluffy.
2. Add coconut milk and vanilla essence. Add almond meal, coconut flour, baking powder substitute and desiccated coconut, combine well.
3. Line a loaf tin with baking paper and poor in coconut mixture.
4. Place in oven for 50-60 minutes or until cooked. Test by inserting a knife into the middle of the loaf.

Chestnut Cake

Ingredients:

600g chestnut flour
3 Tbsp. olive oil
70g raisins
40g pine nuts
40g walnuts
Rosemary

How you make it:

1. Sieve the chestnut flour into a mixing bowl and gradually add 800ml of water, whisking continually to avoid lumps forming, until you have a smooth paste, neither too runny nor too thick, but forming ribbons when it falls from the spoon.
2. Soak the raisins and squeeze out the excess water. Add two T of oil, and then the raisins, pine nuts and shelled walnuts to the batter.
3. Pour the mixture into a shallow, greased baking tray (the cake should only be about 1cm high), sprinkle some rosemary leaves on top and drizzle a Tbsp. of oil over.
4. Put in the oven for thirty minutes. Leave aside for about half an hour before serving, as the cake should be eaten either tepid or cold.

Apple Cinnamon Turnover

Ingredients:

1 medium tart apple, peeled and chopped
1/2 cup applesauce
2 tbsp. Sugar
3/4 tsp ground cinnamon, divided
1 tube (7 1/2 oz.) refrigerated biscuits
1 tbsp. butter or margarine, melted
Dash ground nutmeg

How you make it:

2. In a bowl, combine the apple, applesauce, 1/4 tsp cinnamon and nutmeg.
3. Separate biscuits; roll out each into a 6-in. circle. Place on greased baking sheets, place a heaping tablespoonful of apple mixture in the center of each.
4. Fold in half and pinch edges to seal. Brush with butter.
5. Combine sugar and remaining cinnamon; sprinkle over tops.
6. Bake at 400 degrees for 8-10 minutes or until edges are golden brown. Serve warm.

Favorite Spinach Fritata

Ingredients:

2 hard-boiled eggs
1/2 teaspoon olive oil
2 cups fresh spinach
1 clove garlic, grated

How you make it:

2. Remove stems.
3. Wash the spinach thoroughly in warm salt water. Rinse.
4. Chop coarsely. Cook spinach until it wilts.
5. Beat in garlic and hard-boiled eggs. Heat olive oil, in medium saucepan.
6. Pour in hard-boiled egg mixture. Cook for about two minutes on each side, until hard-boiled egg is firm. Serve.

Broiled Cod with Ginger

Ingredients:

4 - Cod fillets, (1/4 lb. each)
Black pepper (to taste)
1 t grated ginger root or 1/2 tsp. (2 mL) ground ginger
1 1/2 tsp. olive oil
1/4 tsp. paprika

How you make it:

2. Coat a shallow roasting pan with nonstick olive oil.
3. Place cod in pan and sprinkle both sides with pepper and ginger root.
4. Drizzle with oil and sprinkle with paprika.
5. Broil until fish flakes easily with fork, 6-8 minutes.

Salmon and Zucchini Fritters

Ingredients:

2 hard-boiled eggs
1 1/2 cup almond meal
100g freshly cooked salmon, thinly sliced
2 large zucchini, roughly grated, liquid squeezed out
1 Tbsp. chopped dill
Olive oil

How you make it:

1. Combine hard-boiled eggs and almond meal in a bowl and whisk until smooth.
2. Stir with salmon, zucchini, dill and pepper.
3. Place oil in a frying pan and heat over medium heat.
4. Spoon 1 Tbsp. of the salmon mixture into the pan, allowing room for spreading.
5. Cook for 2-3 minutes each side or until golden underneath and cooked through.
6. Remove and repeat with remaining smoked salmon mixture, adding oil to the pan between each batch.

Lime Shrimp

Ingredients:

3 Tbsp. lime juice
1 green onion, chopped
2 Tbsp. chopped cilantro
1 tsp minced, seeded jalapeno peppers
1 tsp. olive oil
1/2 tsp. minced garlic
20 large shrimp (about 1 lb.) peeled and deveined
1 Tbsp. minced red peppers
20 cucumber slices

How you make it:

1. Stir together lime juice, green onion, cilantro, jalapeno peppers, oil and garlic in medium bowl.
2. Toss the shrimp with two T of the dressing in another medium bowl. Cover and refrigerate shrimp for 30 minutes.
3. Preheat broiler or grill. Broil shrimp about 3 inches from heat for 1 1/2 minutes per side or until opaque.
4. Immediately toss hot shrimp with the remaining dressing and red pepper and cool to room temperature. Arrange shrimp on cucumber slices.

Chicken Fast Fingers

Ingredients:

2 boneless skinless chicken breasts, sliced into fingers
1 hard-boiled egg, beaten
1/2 tsp. sea salt
1.5 tsp poultry seasoning
1/2 cup almond flour
1 t dry mustard powder
1/4 - 1/3 cup olive or coconut oil for frying

How you make it:

1. Heat the oil in a large pan over medium heat.
2. Place the beaten hard-boiled egg in one bowl and the almond flour plus seasonings into another bowl.
3. Dip each chicken breast in hard-boiled egg, then in the almond flour mixture.
4. Cook the chicken in two batches until it is golden on each side.

Broccoli with Basil Mushrooms

Ingredients:

1 lbs. frozen broccoli spears
2 Tbsp. olive oil
4-1/2 tsp. basil, chopped
1/3 lbs. whole mushrooms, drained

How you make it:

2. Cook broccoli spears as directed on package. Drain well.
3. Add oil to a saucepan over medium heat. Stir in basil and mushrooms.
4. Cook and stir until thoroughly heated. Spoon over broccoli.

Enjoy

If you Follow through the ultimate guideline provided in The 20/20 Diet B Dr. Phil McGraw , And some of the Healthy and Delicious recipes we hav worked so hard to make for you. You are going to be seeing great results i your body and health, because it is proven to work.

If you enjoyed the recipes in this book, please take the time t share your thoughts and post a positive review with 5 star rating o Amazon, it would encourage us and make us serve you better. It' be greatly appreciated!

If you have any question or anything at all you want to know abou this program, you can hit me up via mail thru jessysmith247@gmail.com I am always there to help you.

Other Health And Fitness Book

The 20/20 Diet: Turn Your Weight Loss Vision Into Reality

Download it Here>> http://www.amazon.com/20-Diet-Weight-Vision-Reality-ebook/dp/B00QMPH9W4

My 10 Day Green Smoothie Cleanse Protein Recipes: 51 Clean Meal Recipes to help you After the 10 Day Smoothie cleanse!

The 10 Days Green Smoothie Cleanse is a Phenomenal Program created to help people lose weight in 10 Days. This program is so powerful and life changing, that lots of people have achieved weight loss.
However, it is sometimes difficult to maintain the weight loss after the 10 day green smoothie cleanse, and that's why we have prepared high-protein meals to Assist with weight loss after the cleanse. In this Book you'll discover lots of High protein recipes that are healthy, clean, and delicious!

Get it HERE>> http://www.amazon.com/Green-Smoothie-Cleanse-Protein-Recipes-ebook/dp/B00KDQZH2C

Get This Bestseller ... My Bulletproof Diet Recipes: Lose up to a Pound a Day, Reclaim Energy and Focus, Upgrade Your Life. Discover delicious Recipes that would help you loss weight were other Diet has failed.

Download here>>
http://www.amazon.com/My-Bulletproof-Diet-Recipes-bulletproof-ebook/dp/B00QV8QRB6

Get this bestselling Green Smoothie Book... **Green Smoothie Recipe Book For Beginners: 10 Day Green Smoothie Cleanse: 51 Essential Gluten-Free, Dairy-Free Green Smoothies to Help You lose Up to 15 Lbs. in 10 Days**
Discover How to get started and Loss 15lbs in 10 Day , Get rid of stubborn body fat, including belly fat, Drop pounds and inches fast, without grueling workouts, live a healthier lifestyle of detoxing and healthy eating
Naturally crave healthy foods so you never have to diet again, and Receive over 50+ All- New recipes for various health conditions and goals.

Click Here Now To Buy>> http://www.amazon.com/Green-Smoothie-Recipe-Book-Beginners-ebook/dp/B00NDLE97S

The Tapping Solution for Weight Loss and Body Confidence is a powerful system that releases the emotions and beliefs that hold us back from loving our bodies. I use tapping on a regular basis and have personally benefitted from this powerful method. It's one of the most important practices in my healing arsenal.

Get The **The Ultimate Tapping Solution Guide: Using EFT to tap your way to WEIGHT LOSS, Wealth and Build Body Confidence for Women**

Click Here>> Amazon U.S Link>> http://www.amazon.com/Ultimate-Tapping-Solution-Guide-Confidence-ebook/dp/B00K6JB97S

Made in the USA
Middletown, DE
30 December 2014